FITNESS FREEDOM FOR SENIORS:

Empowering Elderly Wellness

John Martin

DISCLAIMER

INTRODUCTION

Welcome to "Fitness Freedom for Seniors," a comprehensive program that equips seniors with the knowledge and skills they need to take control of their health and wellbeing. Our meticulously planned exercise programs are meant to increase flexibility, strength, and general vigor. They are changed to take into consideration a range of fitness levels and potential restrictions. Join us as we set out on a path to a healthier, more active lifestyle that will promote independence and self-assurance as you age.

Maintaining excellent health and physical fitness becomes more important as we age. Along with helping to manage weight and avoid chronic diseases, regular exercise and a healthy diet are also important for fostering independence and improving general well-being. The path to

Fitness Freedom for Seniors is encouraging seniors to take charge of their health, break free from inactive routines, and adopt a lifestyle that encourages exercise and a healthy diet.

Join us on our journey to senior fitness freedom if you are a senior citizen looking to improve your overall health, improve fitness, or restore strength and flexibility. Together we will explore the transformative potential of physical activity, embrace healthy eating habits and reap the benefits of an active and rewarding senior life. Regardless of our age, let's bust the myths and take advantage of the freedom fitness brings into our lives.

CHAPTER 1

UNDERSTANDING THE IMPORTANCE OF FITNESS IN SENIORS' LIVES

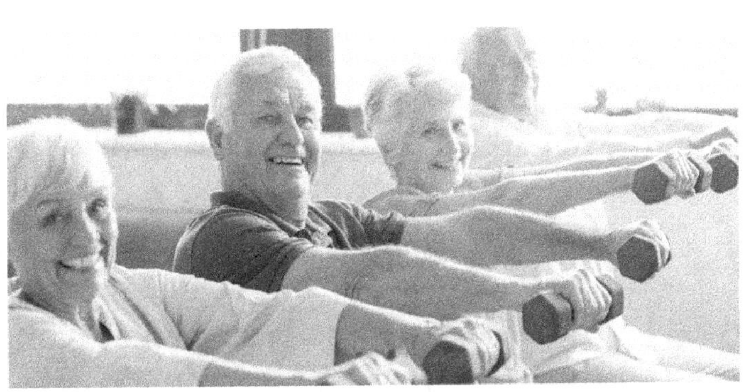

Regardless of age, physical fitness is a crucial part of overall health and well-being. However, for older people, sticking to a regular exercise program becomes even more important. Older people can benefit significantly from regular physical activity in terms of physical, mental and emotional health.

In this section, we explore the value of fitness in the lives of older adults and examine the many benefits of staying active as we age.

- **Physical Health Benefits:**

   The physical health of the elderly can be improved and maintained through regular exercise. Chronic diseases including osteoporosis, osteoarthritis, diabetes and heart disease can be treated with its help. Seniors who exercise regularly can build muscle, increase flexibility and balance, improve their cardiovascular health, and control their weight.

   In addition to strengthening the immune system, exercise reduces the risk of disease and extends life.

- **Mental and Cognitive Benefits:**

The mental and cognitive health of older adults is directly influenced by fitness. Endorphins, or "feel-good" hormones, are released when you exercise, which lowers levels of anxiety, despair and stress. Regular exercise can improve memory, concentration and problem solving while reducing the risk of cognitive decline and diseases such as dementia and Alzheimer's. Exercise promotes brain cell proliferation and improves overall mental health.

- **Social Connections and Emotional Well-being:**

Seniors who participate in physical fitness activities have the opportunity to interact socially and form and maintain relationships. Community fitness classes, walking clubs, and gym visits encourage socialization and interaction, which reduces feelings of isolation and loneliness.

Additionally, training with others creates a sense of support and belonging, which improves overall happiness and emotional health.

- **Disease Prevention and Management:**

Physical exercise has a significant impact on disease prevention and management in the elderly. Regular exercise can help control blood pressure, control cholesterol levels and reduce the risk of heart disease and stroke. It also improves insulin sensitivity, which helps treat diabetes. Exercise strengthens bones, reducing the risk of osteoporosis and fractures. Plus, staying active supports a healthy immune system, making older adults less susceptible to illness and disease

The comprehensive health and well-being of older adults depends on realizing and accepting the value of fitness in their lives. Seniors who prioritize fitness may enjoy better health, happier emotions, lower healthcare costs, and stronger purpose. Accept the idea of "fitness freedom for seniors" and reap the many benefits of leading a healthy lifestyle.

1.2 BENEFITS OF MAINTAINING AN ACTIVE LIFESTYLE

- **Enhancing Physical Health:**

  Regular exercise promotes cardiovascular health, reduces the risk of chronic diseases, including heart disease, diabetes and some malignancies, and helps maintain a healthy weight.

- **Boost Mental Health:**

  Endorphins are natural mood enhancers released during exercise that help reduce tension, anxiety, and depressive symptoms.

- **Enhance Muscle and Bone Strength:**

  The risk of osteoporosis and fractures is reduced through regular physical activity, which includes weight-bearing exercises, which help build and maintain healthy muscles and bones.

- **Reduce Chronic Pain:**

By improving muscle strength and joint flexibility, specific workouts and stretches help treat chronic pain issues like back pain and arthritis.

- **Enhances Cardiovascular Health**:

Aerobic exercises like running, swimming, and cycling strengthen the heart and improve blood circulation, which reduces the risk of cardiovascular disease.

- **Boosts Self-Confidence:**

  Achieving fitness goals and engaging in regular physical activity can improve body image and self-esteem, thereby boosting self-confidence.

- **Increase Longevity:**

  An active lifestyle has been linked to increased life expectancy, as it contributes to overall health and reduces the risk of chronic diseases

Remember that leading an active lifestyle doesn't require intense exercise; many of these advantages can be obtained from even modest activities like brisk strolling. For a lasting, healthy lifestyle, it's crucial to pick things you enjoy and include them in your schedule.

1.3 SECRETS OF HEALTH AND FITNESS:

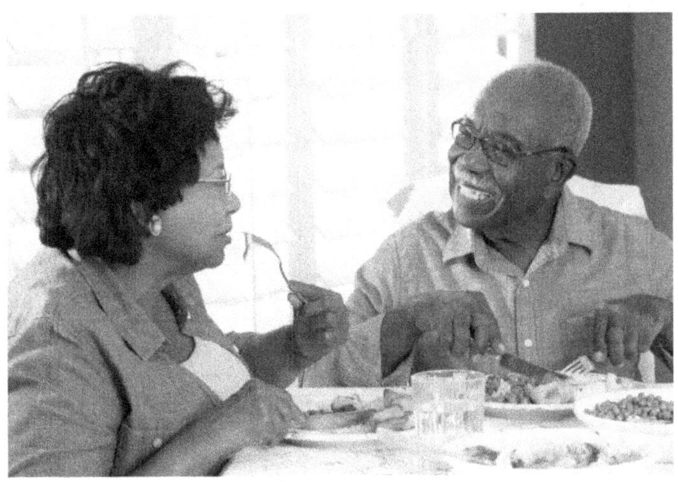

I will reveal to you some secret ways of boosting your health and being fit.

1. Healthy eating

2. Regular exercise

3. Stress management

4. Alternate health and medicine options

5. Sleep well

First and foremost, you should be aware that leading a highly healthy life with an appropriate and healthy lifestyle is necessary for achieving a healthy and fit lifestyle.

You need a few key components to lead a fit and healthy life; without them, you won't be able to achieve the level of health and fitness you desire.

The majority of people believe that they cannot have a healthy and active life unless they adopt a particular tasteless food plan and work hard in the gym, but this is not totally accurate. Exercise and a healthy diet are crucial, but they are not the only things you need to do to keep your health in check.

1. Healthy eating:

Vegetables, fruit, unsaturated fat, and unprocessed carbs are examples of natural ingredients that should be added. You may first find it challenging to include these things in your diet plan, but as you gain more knowledge about the nutritional benefits of various diets, choosing the optimal diet plan will become much simpler for you.

Fast food and junk food should be avoided since they include harmful fat, processed carbohydrates, and other similar ingredients that can be very unhealthy and significantly raise your weight.

2. **Regular Exercise**:

Exercise is another essential factor that you should incorporate into your daily regimen. Some people believe that they will receive a thorough workout program only after joining a gym and paying a high membership fee, but this is untrue. Additionally, individuals today do not have the time to go to the gym every day. Working more than 12 hours a day is necessary to live and succeed in office routines since they are so demanding. You must find a different option at that gym. You can incorporate some brisk walking and jogging into your schedule either in the evening or by rising 25 to 30 minutes earlier than usual and going for a walk.

By using your automobile less, you can also incorporate some walking into your daily routine. You probably use your automobile to get to the grocery store and other common places, but you could walk instead.

3. **Stress Management:**

Another thing that might have a significant positive impact on your life is being free of stress. The stress level can be significantly raised by a hectic work schedule and a lack of downtime, and in many situations, I have witnessed patients develop sleeping disorders as a result of this ongoing stress. You might practice relaxation techniques like yoga or opt for a massage once every two to three weeks to avoid this tension and lessen its consequences.

You may greatly reduce the negative effects of stress by using these techniques, which will also make your life tranquil and stress-free. Your ability to focus on your task and overall productivity will both rise when you are less stressed.

4. **Alternate Health and Medicine Options:**

You should try to stay away from traditional doctors and medications as much as possible because they can have negative impacts on your health. You shouldn't seek out more conventional antibiotics if you have minor health issues like a fever, the flu, or other similar conditions; instead, look for alternative treatments with fewer side effects, such as homeopathy, massage therapy, and other similar techniques.

These techniques will not only help you overcome that health issue, but they are also made entirely of all-natural ingredients, making them even better for your body. You can check into herbal remedies, massage treatments, meditation, Ayurveda, reflexology, and aromatherapy as further complementary and alternative medicine choices.

5.   **Sleep well:**

Another crucial component of your life is sleeping, which is essential for helping your body and mind unwind and prepare for the day's work. If you have trouble sleeping well, take action to improve your situation, since I have witnessed people driving themselves insane because they are unable to get enough rest. You must be careful to avoid bringing work into bed in order to have more rest and better sleep. Make sure you have resolved all of your work and office issues before bed, and if there are any left, put them aside for the evening so you can focus on obtaining a good night's sleep

Some people make an effort to follow good diet and exercise plans, but they usually only stick with them for brief periods of time. Because you need to be highly constant for optimal effects, this is also not very successful. This is the reason

I've included some actions that are quite
simple to take and that you can keep up
with in any situation.

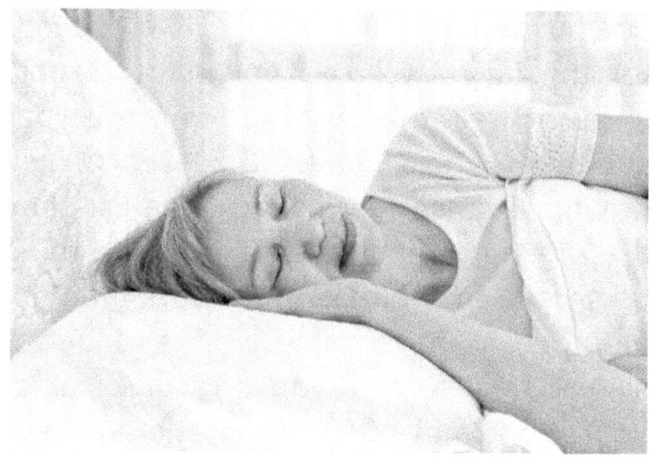

CHAPTER 2

ASSESSING YOUR CURRENT FITNESS LEVEL

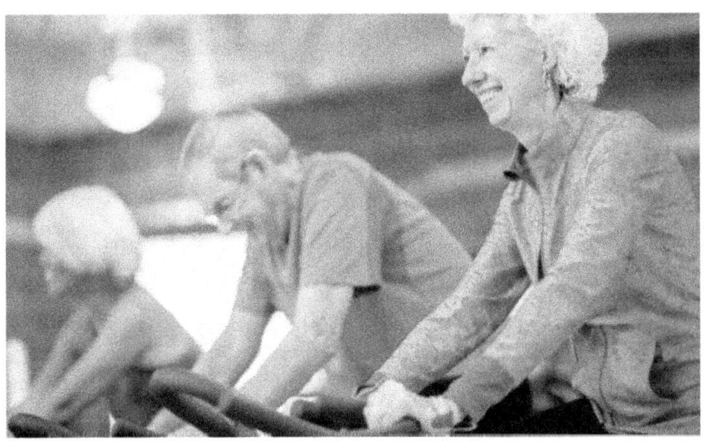

You must promise yourself that you will improve your life, and you must then honor that promise with all of your might. Making a personalized fitness plan that fits your objectives and capabilities requires an accurate assessment of your current level of fitness. Making a personalized fitness plan that fits your objectives and capabilities requires an accurate assessment of your current level of fitness.

- **Cardiovascular Endurance:**

  Cardiovascular endurance refers to the ability of the heart, lungs and blood vessels to deliver oxygen to the muscles during prolonged physical activity. To measure this, you can do a 12-minute run/walk test (measure the distance you walk in 12 minutes) or a 1-mile walk test. These tests assess your aerobic capacity and provide insight into your current level of cardiovascular fitness.

- **Muscular Strength and Endurance:**

  Having strong and durable muscles is essential for general fitness. Push-ups, sit-ups, and one-repetition maximum (1RM) tests for certain exercises like the bench press or squat can all be used to evaluate your strength. Your muscular endurance can be determined by keeping track of how many repetitions you can complete with proper form and a given weight. By using this evaluation to identify your strengths and weaknesses, you can adjust your exercise regimen.

Having strong and durable muscles is essential for general fitness. Push-ups, sit-ups, and one-repetition maximum (1RM) tests for certain exercises like the bench press or squat can all be used to evaluate your strength. Your muscular endurance can be determined by keeping track of how many repetitions you can complete with proper form and a given weight. By using this evaluation to identify your strengths and weaknesses, you can adjust your exercise regimen

- **Flexibility:**

Maintaining joint mobility and avoiding injuries require flexibility. Exercises like the sit-and-reach test, in which you measure how far you can reach while sitting with your legs straight, can be used to determine your flexibility.

This exercise measures how flexible your hamstrings and lower back are. The hip rotation test and the shoulder flexibility test are further techniques. You can include particular stretching exercises in your program by locating your tight spots.

- **Body Composition:**

Maintaining In order to evaluate your general health and fitness, it is essential to understand your body composition, specifically your ratio of lean muscle mass to body fat. This can be accomplished using a variety of techniques, including dual-energy x-ray absorptiometry

(DEXA) scans, bioelectrical impedance, and skinfold measures. These examinations measure the distribution of muscle and fat across your body.

Monitoring your body composition enables you to assess how well you're doing with your efforts to lose weight or increase muscle. Joint mobility and avoiding injuries require flexibility. Exercises like the sit-and-reach test, in which you measure how far you can reach while sitting with your legs straight, can be used to determine your flexibility. This exercise measures how flexible your hamstrings and lower back are. The hip rotation test and the shoulder flexibility test are further techniques. You can include particular stretching exercises in your program by locating your tight spots.

In order to evaluate your general health and fitness, it is essential to understand your body composition, specifically your ratio of lean muscle mass to body fat. This can be accomplished using a variety of techniques, including dual-energy x-ray absorptiometry (DEXA) scans, bioelectrical impedance, and skinfold measures.

These examinations measure the distribution of muscle and fat across your body. Monitoring your body composition enables you to assess how well you're doing with your efforts to lose weight or increase muscle.

2.1 Self-Evaluation: Physical Abilities and Limitations

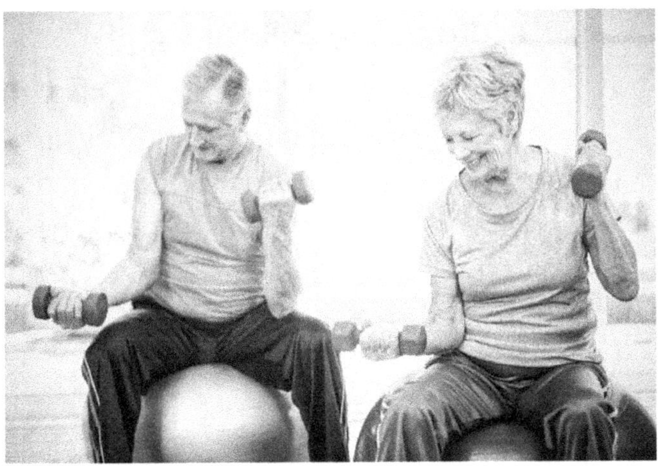

I will evaluate my physical capabilities, weaknesses, and strengths in this self-evaluation. Understanding these factors is essential for maintaining a healthy lifestyle and setting realistic goals.

Physical Abilities

- **Cardiovascular Fitness:**

  I regularly do cardiovascular exercise like jogging and cycling which has improved my endurance and heart health. I can now comfortably complete a 5km run without excessive fatigue.

- **Strength:**

  I will evaluate my physical capabilities, weaknesses, and strengths in this self-evaluation. Understanding these factors is essential for maintaining a healthy lifestyle and setting realistic goals. My overall muscle strength has increased as a result of consistent strength training sessions. I can now exercise with my body weight and lift heavier weights with better form and control.

- **Balance and Coordination:**

I will evaluate my physical capabilities, weaknesses, and strengths in this self-evaluation. Understanding these factors is essential for maintaining a healthy lifestyle and setting realistic goals. My overall muscle strength has increased as a result of consistent strength training sessions. I can now exercise with my body weight and lift heavier weights with better form and control.

My coordination and balance have improved thanks to exercises like yoga and balance-focused workouts. I have more stability in my stances and can execute difficult motions.

- **Flexibility:**

Regular yoga practice and stretching exercises have improved my flexibility. I can now stretch in a variety of ways with more comfort and less pain.

Physical Limitations

- **Time Constraints:**

  Sometimes I can only spend a short amount of time exercising due to my hectic job schedule. My exercise regimen has occasionally been inconsistent as a result of this.

- **Injury History:**

  Running is one of the high-impact activities that occasionally makes my old knee injury hurt. I've chosen lower-impact exercises because of this restriction to avoid putting myself under additional strain.

- **Flexibility Restrictions:**

  Despite my progress, I still encounter certain flexibility restrictions in several areas. This interferes with my ability to execute some yoga poses properly.

This self-assessment has provided valuable insight into my physical abilities and limitations. By recognizing strengths and areas for improvement, I'm better able to adjust my fitness routine and make informed decisions to live a healthier lifestyle.

2.3 Medical Considerations and Consultations

Despite my progress, I still encounter certain flexibility restrictions in several areas. This interferes with my ability to execute some yoga poses properly.

Medical Consideration:

- **Allergies:**

  I am allergic to shellfish and certain types of nuts. While these allergies haven't caused any significant issues in training, it's important to be careful with my diet and what supplements I may choose to take.

- **Pre-existing Conditions:**

  I've had asthma in the past, which can occasionally make it difficult for me to perform demanding aerobic workouts. During workouts, I need to be cautious and make sure my inhaler is close by.

- **Medications:**

  I presently take a daily hypertension medicine. This necessitates regular monitoring of my blood pressure and checking to make sure that my workout regimen does not negatively impact the medicine.

Medical Consultation:

- **Consulting a Physician:**

  It's imperative to talk to my primary care physician before beginning any new workout program or making any adjustments to my daily routine. Given my current medical issues and treatment plan, this is very crucial.

- **Tailored Recommendations:**

  A medical professional may give me individualized guidance on the level, length, and kind of exercise that is best for my particular health needs. They can also provide advice on how to handle any hazards that might be connected to my medical conditions.

- **Monitoring and Adjustments:**

  A medical professional may give me individualized guidance on the level, length, and kind of exercise that is best for my particular health needs. They can also provide advice on how to handle any hazards that might be connected to my medical conditions.

Maintaining a safe and efficient workout routine requires an understanding of and attention to my medical needs. I may strive toward my health and fitness goals while reducing potential dangers to my wellbeing by getting medical counsel and adhering to a plan that is well-informed.

2.3 SETTING REALISTIC FITNESS GOALS

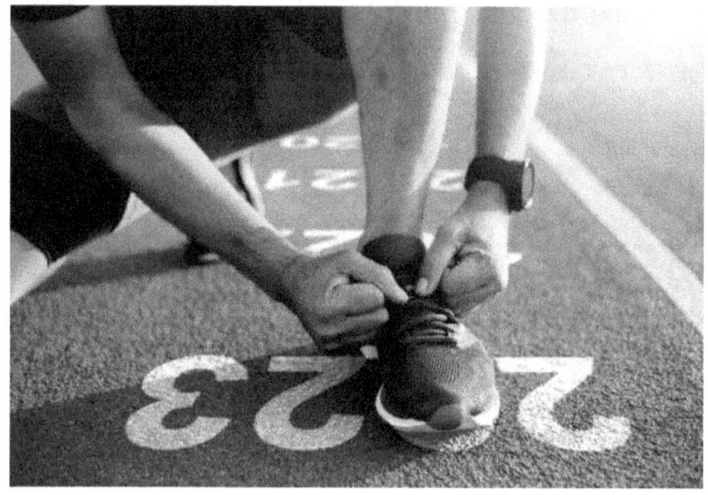

In this section, I will discuss the importance of setting realistic fitness goals and provide a framework for setting achievable goals that align with my current level of fitness, lifestyle, and long-term aspirations.

Understanding Realistic Goals

- **Assessing Current Fitness:**

  Before setting goals, it is important to have a clear idea of my current level of fitness. This includes the assessment of strengths, weaknesses and any limitations, such as e.g. B. medical considerations or time constraints.

- **Smart Criteria:**

  Specific, measurable, achievable, relevant, and time-bound (SMART) goals should be set. With this framework, success is more likely because goals are well-defined and attainable.

Type of Goals

- **Short-term Goals:**

  These can be achieved in a few weeks to a few months. For example, I want to increase the number of push-ups I can do in a minute or run 0.5 km more in a month.

- **Medium-term Goals:**

  They can be completed in three to six months. For example, losing a certain amount of weight, completing 10,000 runs, or reducing your body fat percentage.

- **Long-term Goals:**

These are overarching goals that may take a year or more to achieve. Long-term goals might include running a marathon, achieving a major weight loss goal, or mastering advanced yoga poses.

Factors to be Considered

- **Realistic Progression:**

Goals should be ambitious but achievable. Goals that are too ambitious can lead to burnout or disappointment, while goals that are too easy may not give a sense of accomplishment.

- **Time Commitment:**

  Consider the time available for training and the frequency of training sessions. Avoid setting goals that require more time and effort than you can reasonably invest.

- **Health Consideration:**

  Consider any previous illnesses or physical limitations. Goals should support overall health and well-being.

Tracking Progress:

- **Measurements and Data:**

  Track relevant stats like weight, body measurements, fitness test results, and exercise frequency. This data helps to objectively evaluate progress.

- **Adjustment and Flexibility:**

  Be open to adjusting goals based on actual progress. If progress is slower or faster than expected, it's important to adjust your goals accordingly.

- **Setting realistic fitness goals:**

  It's an essential step to achieving long-term success and staying motivated. By following the SMART criteria and taking into account personal factors, I can set goals that actually improve my fitness journey and ultimately lead to a healthier, more active lifestyle.

CHAPTER 3

FOUNDATION OF SENIOR FITNESS

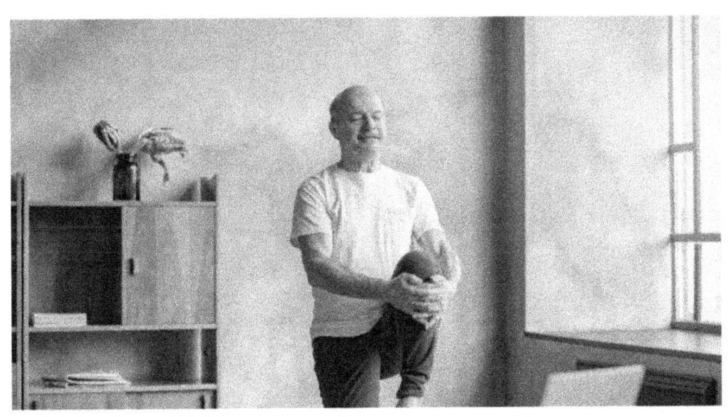

Promoting health, functional ability, and quality of life as people age is the cornerstone of senior fitness. It entails specialized workout plans that target physical restrictions, place an emphasis on functional motions, and promote cardiovascular, muscular, and skeletal health.

For the purpose of maintaining independence in daily tasks, flexibility, strength, and balance are given priority. Customization, slow progression, and ongoing evaluation guarantee security and efficiency. A comprehensive approach to elder exercise emphasizes social involvement and general wellbeing as vital components.

3.1 THE PILLARS OF FITNESS:
Endurance, Strength, Balance, Flexibility

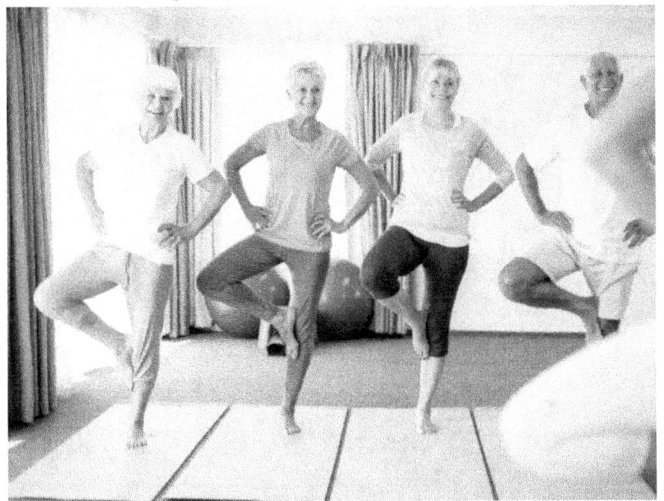

The idea of fitness entails a comprehensive strategy that takes into account various facets of physical health. The fundamental elements that make up the four pillars of fitness—endurance, strength, balance, and flexibility—contribute to general health and functionality. Each pillar contributes in a different way to maintaining an active and healthy lifestyle.

- **Endurance**:

The focus of endurance, commonly referred to as cardiovascular fitness, is the body's capacity to maintain sustained physical activity. To effectively provide oxygen and nutrients to the muscles, the circulatory and respiratory systems must function properly. Exercises like walking, jogging, swimming, or cycling aid in increasing lung capacity, improving heart health, and increasing endurance levels. Increased stamina, a lower risk of developing chronic diseases, and improved weight management are all benefits of endurance exercise.

- **Strength**:

Strength is the basis of physical strength and functional ability. It involves the ability of muscles to exert force against resistance. Strength training, through activities such as weight lifting, bodyweight exercises, and resistance bands, helps build muscle mass, bone density, and overall strength.

The increase in strength supports daily activities, maintains correct posture and improves metabolism. Strong muscles also contribute to joint stability, reducing the risk of injury.

- **Balance**:

The ability of the body to maintain equilibrium and avoid falling is known as balance, and it becomes increasingly important as we age. It depends on how the neurological and muscular systems communicate with one another. Exercises for maintaining equilibrium include standing on one leg, performing yoga positions, and using stability balls. Enhancing balance increases proprioception, lowers the chance of falling, and improves agility and coordination.

- **Flexibility**:

Flexibility refers to the range of motion around a joint. This is the elasticity of muscles, tendons and ligaments. Regular stretching and flexibility exercises, such as static and dynamic stretching, yoga, and Pilates, help maintain and improve mobility.

Adequate flexibility prevents muscle imbalances, supports joint mobility and reduces the risk of injury. It also helps maintain good posture and allows for smoother movements.

The four fitness pillars of endurance, strength, balance, and flexibility work in concert to produce a holistic strategy for physical well-being. Holistic health, functional abilities, and a higher quality of life are all supported by a well-rounded fitness regimen that includes exercises from each of these pillars. A well-rounded and lasting fitness journey that meets the many needs of the human body is possible when all four areas are worked on to a high level of competency.

3.2 TAILORING YOUR FITNESS ROUTINE

To achieve real, long-lasting success in your fitness, you must design a regimen that fits your unique demands. Your goals, level of fitness, tastes, and any potential limits should all be taken into account while designing your regimen. This individualized method optimizes efficiency and fun while lowering the danger of harm.

- **Identify Your Goals:**

  Establish your fitness objectives first. Are you trying to lose weight, grow muscle, enhance cardiovascular health, increase flexibility, or do all of the above? You can plan your routine effectively by expressing your goals clearly.

- **Assess Your Current Fitness Level:**

  Honest self-evaluation is essential. Take into account your present level of fitness, your strengths and weaknesses, as well as any medical restrictions or physical limits. You can use this information to help you choose the right exercises and prevent overexertion.

- **Choose Activities You Enjoy:**

  Take part in things you actually enjoy doing. The possibility of consistency rises when anything is enjoyable, whether it be dancing, swimming, hiking, or playing a sport. Find ways to add exercise to your regimen that you enjoy.

- **Consider Time Commitment:**

  Determine how much time you can actually spend exercising. Both the length of each workout and the number of days per week you may devote are taken into consideration. A healthy habit fits into your schedule without putting you under pressure.

- **Balance Cardiovascular and Strength Training:**

  Incorporate both cardiovascular (aerobic) exercises and strength training. Cardio boosts your heart health and burns calories, while strength training builds muscle and increases metabolism. Balance these components based on your goals.

- **Include Flexibility and Balance Exercises:**

  Don't overlook flexibility and balance exercises. Stretching and balance work enhance joint mobility, reduce the risk of injuries, and support functional movements in daily life.

- **Listen to Your Body:**

  Keep track of how your body responds to various exercises. If something hurts or makes you uncomfortable, change it or don't do it. To prevent overtraining, take breaks as needed.

- **Seek Professional Guidance:**

  Consider speaking with a fitness expert if you're new to training, have special objectives, or need to work around medical issues. They can assist in creating a regimen that is safe and meets your needs.

3.3 THE ROLE OF NUTRITION AND HYDRATION in SENIOR FITNESS

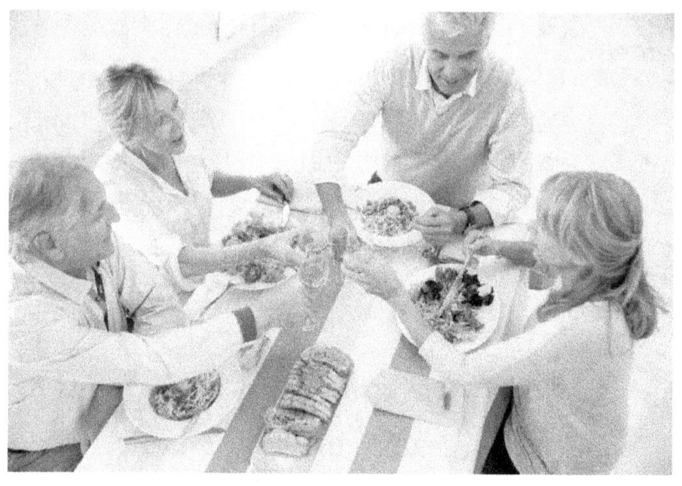

Senior fitness depends heavily on nutrition and hydration, which also have a big impact on general health, energy levels, and physical performance. Age-related changes in the body's nutritional requirements make it more important than ever for seniors to maintain an active and fulfilling lifestyle.

- **Adequate Nutrient Intake:**

  A balanced diet that includes important elements including

protein, carbs, healthy fats, vitamins, and minerals is necessary for seniors. Protein is crucial for supporting tissue regeneration, preserving muscular mass, and keeping muscles strong.

- **Bone Health:**

For preserving bone health and avoiding osteoporosis, calcium and vitamin D are essential nutrients. Bone strength is improved by consuming enough dairy products, leafy greens, fortified foods, and sunlight.

- **Hydration:**

All ages need to be well hydrated, but seniors need it even more because their ability to feel thirst is diminished. Fatigue, diminished cognitive function, and urinary tract problems can all result from dehydration. Regular water

consumption is essential, as are
hydrating foods like fruits and
soups.

- **Fiber for Digestion:**

  Whole grains, fruits, and vegetables
  are examples of foods high in fiber
  that help with digestion, reduce
  constipation, and support a
  balanced gut microbiota.

- **Avoid Empty Calories:**

  Limiting added sugars and
  processed carbs lowers the risk of
  diabetes and cardiovascular
  disease, stabilizes blood sugar
  levels, and helps prevent weight
  gain.

- **Medication and Nutrition
  Interaction:**

  Seniors who use medicine should be
  mindful of any possible interactions
  with particular foods. Negative

interactions can be prevented by seeking the advice of a healthcare expert.

- **Customized Diet Plans:**

  Developing a personalized nutrition plan that addresses the needs of senior fitness requires careful consideration of each person's dietary choices, food allergies, and any underlying medical concerns.

- **Mindful Eating:**

  Paying attention to hunger and fullness signals while eating might help you avoid overeating and foster a positive relationship with food.

Senior fitness depends on proper nutrition and hydration to promote physical health, energy levels, and general wellbeing. Seniors can maintain their immune system, muscle mass, and bone health with the support of a balanced diet full of important nutrients and adequate hydration. Individualized recommendations for the best nutrition and hydration can be obtained by speaking with a healthcare provider or certified dietitian.

CHAPTER 4

CARDIOVASCULAR HEALTH AND ENDURANCE

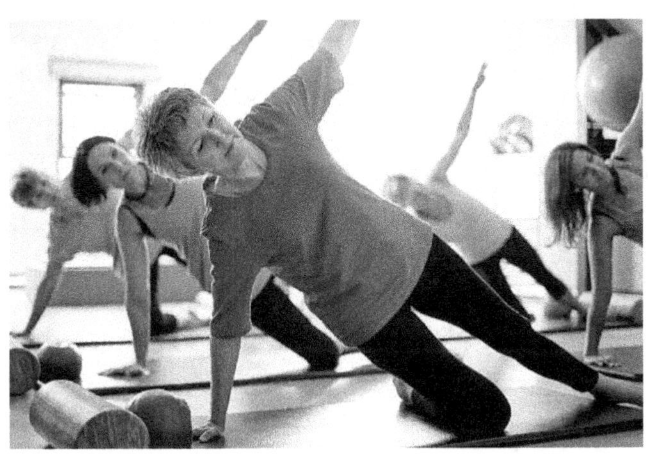

The condition of the heart, blood vessels, and circulatory system is referred to as cardiovascular health. It is crucial for the body to function at its best because the heart transports waste and supplies nutrition and oxygen to the body's organs.

Contrarily, endurance describes the body's capacity to maintain physical activity for an extended period of time without becoming exhausted. The capacity of the heart and lungs to provide oxygen-rich blood to the muscles while engaging in physical activity is known as cardiovascular endurance.

For general fitness and well-being, having strong cardiovascular health and endurance is essential. Regular aerobic workouts, such as walking, jogging, swimming, or cycling, strengthen the heart and improve blood circulation, both of which help to improve cardiovascular health.

Regular exercise also helps to regulate body weight, cut cholesterol, enhance blood pressure, and improve respiratory function. It can reduce the chance of developing cardiovascular conditions like high blood pressure, heart disease, and stroke.

4.1 CHOOSING THE RIGHT CARDIO EXERCISES FOR SENIORS

Choosing the right cardio exercises for seniors is crucial for maintaining their overall health and well-being. Regular physical activity can improve cardiovascular health, increase endurance, and help manage weight. However, it is important to take into consideration the limitations and health conditions that may be specific to seniors when selecting appropriate exercises.

Here are some factors to consider when choosing cardio exercises for seniors:

- **Low Impact Exercises:**

  Joint health becomes more crucial as we get older. Choose low-impact exercises like walking, swimming, cycling, or using elliptical machines over high-impact ones that strain the joints. Because these workouts are easy on the joints, there is less chance of harm or aggravation of current joint diseases like arthritis.

- **Proper warm-up and cool-down:**

  Warm up before each workout session to get the body ready for movement and lower the risk of injury. This can be done by gently moving, stretching out slightly, or marching in place.

  Similarly, include a cool-down break at the end of each session to let the body recuperate and progressively lower the heart rate. This can involve gradual, gentle motions and stretches.

- **Gradual progression:**

  Seniors should begin their workouts with activities that are appropriate for their present level of fitness and progressively increase the intensity and duration as they go. This prevents strain or overexertion and enables the body to adapt. A safe and efficient workout program can be created with the help of a healthcare expert or a certified fitness trainer.

- **Safety considerations:**

When choosing aerobic workouts for seniors, safety should come first. It's crucial to wear the right shoes, drink plenty of water, and work out in a place that is well-lit and secure. Before beginning any new fitness program, seniors with particular medical ailments or concerns should speak with their healthcare professional

- **Enjoyment:**

It is crucial to find cardio exercises that seniors enjoy and are motivated to continue regularly. This can include activities like dancing, gardening, playing tennis, or even joining group exercise classes. Enjoyment increases adherence, making it more likely that seniors will stick to their exercise routine.

4.2 CARDIOVASCULAR WORKOUTS FOR DIFFERENT FITNESS LEVELS

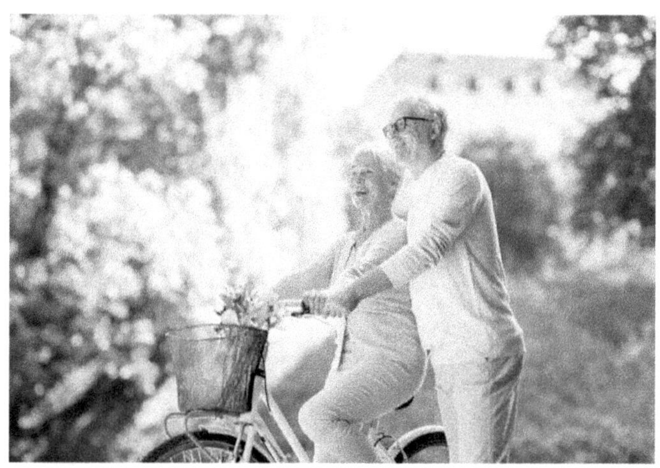

Sure, I'd be pleased to offer you some advice on cardiovascular exercises for various fitness levels:

BEGINNERS:

- **Brisk Walking:** Start by going for a 20 to 30 minute walk at a pace that raises your heart rate while still enabling you to speak.

- **Cycling**: Then, try riding for 15-20 minutes at a relaxed speed on level ground.

- **Jumping Jacks:** Perform 3 sets of 20 jumping jacks with short breaks in between.

- **Dance Workout:** For 15-20 minutes, adhere to a beginner-level dance training video.

IMMEDIATE:

- **Running or Jogging:** Start with a 10-15 minute jog, then for 20–30 minutes alternate between 1-2 minutes of jogging and 1-2 minutes of walking.

- **Interval Training:**

  For 20 to 25 minutes, alternate between 3 minutes of low-intensity exercise (such as jumping rope) and 1 minute of high-intensity activity (such as sprinting or quick burgees).

- **Swimming**:

  Swim laps for 20-30 minutes, alternating between freestyle and a slower stroke to recover.

- **Circuit Training:**

  Perform a circuit of bodyweight exercises for 30 seconds each, pausing for 15 seconds in between sets of pushups, squats, lunges, and burpees. Circulate three to four times.

- **High-Intensity Interval Training (HIIT):**

  Sprinting, kettlebell swings, and box jumps are a few examples of strenuous exercises that you can practice for 40 seconds each, followed by a 20-second break. Continue for 4-5 sets.

- **Running Interval:**

  Run at a fast pace for 2 minutes, followed by 1 minute of recovery jogging. Repeat this pattern for 20-25 minutes.

- **Indoor Cycling:**

  A high-intensity spin class might be worth trying, or you could design your own interval workout with a range of resistance and speed.

- **Rowing**:

  Row at a high intensity for 500 meters, then rest for 1-2 minutes. Repeat for 4-5 sets.

Each workout should begin with a warm-up and end with a cool-down. To prevent damage, always pay attention to your body and gradually increase the duration and intensity of your workouts. Before beginning a new exercise regimen, it's a good idea to speak with a fitness expert or healthcare provider, especially if you have any underlying medical issues.

4.3 MONITORING HEART RATE AND INTENSITY SAFELY

Seniors must keep an eye on their heart rate and intensity during cardiac exercises to maintain their safety and wellbeing. The main considerations are outlined in the following list:

- **Check your pulse or use a heart rate monitor:**

  Seniors should periodically check their heart rates when exercising using a heart rate monitor or by manually taking their pulse. They are able to avoid overexertion and maintain their desired heart rate range thanks to this.

- **Work out the target heart rate zone:**

  Seniors should figure out their target heart rate zone depending on their age, level of fitness, and any pre-existing medical issues. This range helps to maximize the cardiovascular benefits while ensuring that the workout intensity is adequate.

- **Gradually upping intensity:**

Seniors should start out mild and then gradually up the intensity over time. This lowers the possibility of unexpected heart rate increases and enables the body to respond.

- **Pay attention to your body:**

Seniors should pay attention to how their bodies feel while exercising. They must refrain from exerting themselves to the point of severe exhaustion or discomfort. They should stop exercising and, if required, seek medical assistance if they feel chest pain, dizziness, or shortness of breath.

- **Drink plenty of water:**

  To maintain healthy cardiac function and avoid dehydration, seniors should drink plenty of water before, during, and after activity. It is advised to drink water throughout the workout.

- **Speak with a medical expert:**

  Seniors with particular health ailments or worries should speak with their doctor before beginning or changing an exercise plan. They might include recommendations and best practices for secure heart rate monitoring during activity.

By monitoring heart rate and intensity safely, seniors can ensure that their cardio exercises are effective and safe. Regular monitoring helps seniors optimize cardiovascular benefits, avoid overexertion, and exercise within their safe fitness limits.

CHAPTER 5

BUILDING STRENGTH SAFELY

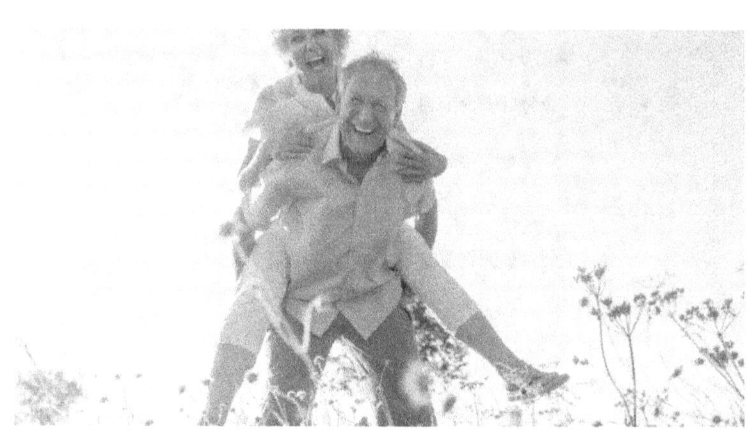

Safe strength development is crucial for avoiding accidents and ensuring steady advancement. Here is a thorough manual on how to increase strength while putting safety first:

- **Establish Correct Form First:**

    Prior to increasing weight or intensity, concentrate on perfecting the proper form for each exercise. The danger of injury is reduced, and the right muscle groups are targeted when you use proper technique.

- **Warm-up:**

  Perform a dynamic warm-up before strength training that incorporates motions that resemble the workouts you'll be doing. This improves blood flow, warms up your muscles, and gets your body ready for the workout that will soon begin.

- **Gradual Progression:**

  Start with lesser weights and progressively boost the resistance as your muscles get used to it. Avoid the urge to lift high weights too quickly because this can result in sprains and other injuries.

- **Balanced Routine:**

  Design a strength training program that evenly targets each of the main muscle groups. Certain muscles can go neglected, which can result in imbalances and possible injury.

- **Rest and Recovery:**

  Give your muscles enough time between workouts to heal. For each muscle group, aim for at least 48 hours between workouts.

- **Use Spotters and Safety Equipment:**

  When performing exercises like the bench press or squats with large weights, use spotters. In the event that you are unable to complete a lift, safety tools like power cages and safety bars can also act as a safety net.

- **Breathing Technique:**

  It's important to breathe correctly. Before lifting, inhale, and while exerting yourself, exhale. Blood pressure can rise if you hold your breath while lifting.

- **Recovery strategies:**

  To speed up recovery and avoid muscular soreness, combine foam rolling, stretching, and enough sleep after your workout.

- **Avoid overtraining**:

  Injury and burnout can result from excessive training without sufficient rest. Incorporate rest days and lighter weeks into your schedule to allow for healing.

- **Progress Monitoring:**

    Keep a training log to keep tabs on your development. You may track your progress and make any adjustments to your regimen by keeping track of your lifts, sets, and reps.

It takes perseverance, consistency, and a dedication to using the right form to build strength safely. You can reap the advantages of improved strength while lowering your risk of accidents by adhering to these recommendations.

5.1 UNDERSTANDING AGE-RELATED MUSCLE CHANGES

Age-related muscle changes, also known as sarcopenia, refer to the gradual loss of muscle mass, strength, and function that occurs with aging. These changes can have significant effects on an individual's overall health and physical performance. Here are some key aspects to understanding age-related muscle changes:

- **Loss of muscle mass:**

  The size and quantity of muscle fibers decrease with aging. As a result, muscular mass declines. Around the age of 30, this loss of muscle mass starts, and it picks up speed after the age of 60.

- **Decreased muscular strength:**

  As people get older, their muscular mass also decreases, which contributes to a drop in muscle strength. A person's general quality of life may be impacted by a loss of muscle strength, which can also affect physical function and the risk of falling.

- **Alterations to Muscle Quality:**

In addition to the loss of muscle mass and strength, changes to muscle quality also occur. Included in this are alterations in muscle structure, such as a rise in fat infiltration and connective tissue, which can further support muscular growth.

- **Sedentary Lifestyle:**

Sedentary behavior, which is typical of older persons, might exacerbate the aging-related muscle alterations. Lack of regular exercise and physical activity can hasten muscle loss and exacerbate muscle weakness.

- **Impact of Chronic Illnesses:** Age-related muscle alterations can also be made worse by chronic illnesses like diabetes, heart disease, and arthritis. Inactivity, inflammation, and the breakdown of muscle protein can all be caused by these disorders.

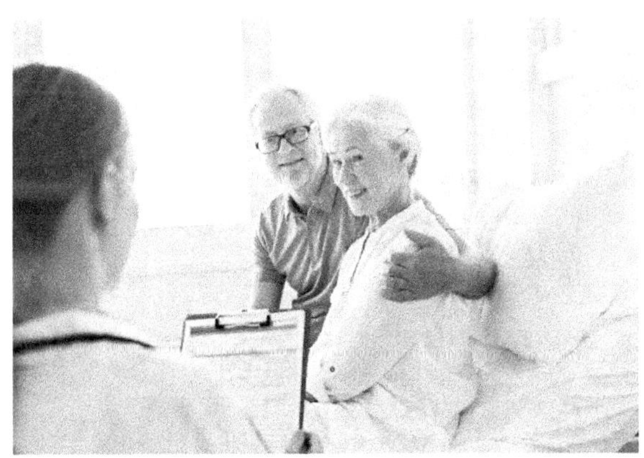

5.2 RESISTANCE TRAINING: BODYWEIGHT, BANDS, WEIGHTS

Working against an opposing force to build muscle strength and tone is known as resistance training. Bodyweight, resistance bands, or weights can all be used, and each has its own advantages.

- **Bodyweight Resistance Training**:

  Workouts using only your body weight are known as bodyweight exercises. Push-ups, squats, lunges, and planks are a few examples. These workouts may be customized to different fitness levels, are convenient, and require little to no equipment.

- **Resistance Bands:**

  When stretched, resistance bands are elastic bands that offer resistance. They are appropriate for people of all fitness levels because they have varied resistance levels. Bands are particularly useful for home exercises while traveling and can be used to target specific muscle groups and increase flexibility.

- **Weight Resistance Training:**

  During weight training, resistance is produced by employing external weights such as machines, barbells, or dumbbells. Progressive overload is possible with this technique, where you gradually raise the weight to put the muscles to the test. Building strength, muscular mass, and bone density with weights is helpful.

5.3 DESIGNING A STRENGTH TRAINING PROGRAM

Designing an effective strength training program involves careful planning to target specific muscle groups, promote progressive overload, and ensure balanced workouts. Here's a comprehensive guide to help you design a well-rounded strength training program:

- **Clear Your Goals:**

  Decide on your objectives, whether they are to increase strength, improve general fitness, or focus on a particular area. Your objectives will affect the type, quantity, and frequency of your exercises.

- **Select Exercises:**

  Choose a range of workouts that target various muscle groups, both complex (multi-joint) and isolated (single-joint). Bench presses, rows, squats, and deadlifts are examples of compound exercises. Bicep curls, tricep extensions, and leg extensions are examples of isolation exercises.

- **Select a training period:**
Determine how frequently you'll exercise each week. Beginners might begin with 2-3 weekly sessions, while more seasoned users might aim for 4-6 weekly sessions. Between strenuous workouts, give your muscles at least one day to heal.

- **Make a split routine:** To prevent overtraining and allow for appropriate recuperation, divide your workouts across the various muscle groups. Full body, upper/lower body, and push/pull/legs are examples of common splits. Pick a split that fits with your schedule and goals.

- **Decide how many repetitions (reps) and sets to perform for each exercise:** Use heavier weights and fewer repetitions (3-6 reps for 3-5 sets) to increase strength. Use moderate weights and moderate rep ranges (8–12 reps for 3–4 sets) to promote hypertrophy (muscle growth).

- **Progressive overload**

  Should be implemented by progressively raising the weight, reps, or sets over time. Strength and muscle gain are stimulated by this. To keep track of your development and modifications, keep a workout journal.

- Include an active warm-up to get your muscles and joints ready for the activity. Then, cool down afterward. Static stretches should be performed after your workout to increase flexibility and lessen discomfort.

- **Rest periods**:

  Take a break in between sets to let your muscles recuperate. longer rest (2–3 minutes) for strength and shorter rest (30–60 seconds) for hypertrophy

- **Nutrition and Hydration:**

  Fuel your body with proper nutrition and stay hydrated. Protein is crucial for muscle repair and growth.

- **Recovery**:

  Give recovery top priority by getting enough sleep, foam rolling, and engaging in light activities on rest days. For the development of muscles and general health, recovery is crucial.

- **Consistency:**

  Consistency is essential for obtaining results. Maintain your plan and make small, steady alterations. Remember that every person has different needs, so think about working with a fitness expert or personal trainer to develop a program that is customized to your unique objectives, level of fitness, and any health issues.

CHAPTER 6

ENHANCING BALANCE AND STABILITY

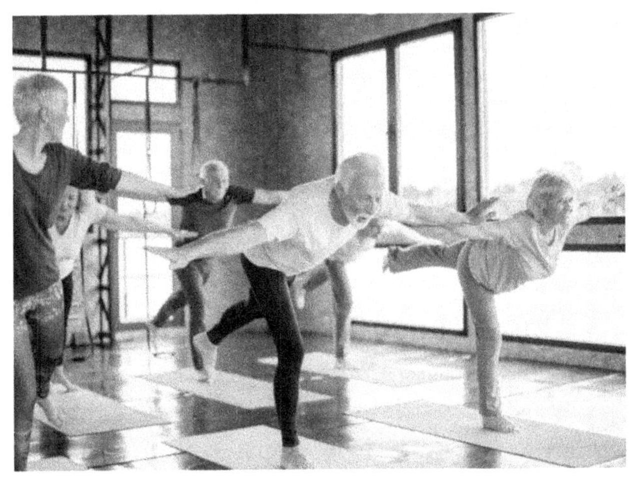

For overall fitness and injury prevention, improving balance and stability is crucial. Coordination, posture, and functional strength can all be improved by incorporating exercises and routines that test your balance and stability. Here are some tips for improving your stability and balance:

- **Balance workouts:**

  Include balance-testing workouts in your routine. Examples include heel-to-toe walking, single-legged standing, and yoga positions like Warrior III and Tree Pose. The stabilizing muscles are worked during these activities, which also enhance proprioception (knowledge of your body's position in space).

- **Work With A Stability Ball:**

  Squats, bridges, and planks are all exercises that can be performed with a stability ball. These exercises demand control and balance while working your core and other stabilizing muscles.

- **Proprioceptive Training:**

  Involves exercises performed on unsteady surfaces like foam pads or balance boards. Your body is

continually forced to change due to
these tools, which improve stability
and balance.

- **Functional Training**:

  Include motions that represent
  everyday activities. When your
  body adjusts to different demands,
  movements like lunges, step-ups,
  and lifting weights unevenly test
  your stability.

- **Strengthening The Core:**

  A stable body is a result of a strong
  core. Target various core muscles
  with exercises including planks, side
  planks, and Russian twists.

- **Pilates And Yoga:**

  Balance, stability, and flexibility are
  stressed in techniques like yoga and

Pilates. Through deliberate movements and poses, they assist in enhancing body awareness and control.

- **Progressive Training:**

Progressively make the balance exercises harder. As your talents advance, move from stable surfaces to unstable ones. Exercise your balance while paying attention to your movements and using your mind. Control and steadiness can be enhanced by mindfulness.

- **Exercises For The Feet And Ankles**:

Stability is improved by having strong feet and ankles. To increase lower body stability, practice calf lifts, ankle circles, and toe taps.

- **Including Unilateral Exercises:**

To correct imbalances and enhance stability on both sides of your body, include unilateral exercises such as single-arm or single-leg exercises in your program.

- **Breathing Methods:**

Useful breathing methods can aid in the stabilization of your body. When practicing balance, pay special attention to your regulated, rhythmic breathing.

- **Regular Practice:**

Balance and stability may be improved with regular practice, just like any other skill. Aim to incorporate balance training into your schedule a couple times per week.

Keep in mind that training for stability and balance is progressive. Start with exercises that are appropriate for your present skill level and gradually increase them as your confidence grows. Before starting a new workout routine, speak with a fitness expert or healthcare provider if you have any current medical ailments or concerns.

6.1 IMPORTANCE OF BALANCE IN FALL PREVENTION

For seniors in particular, who may be more prone to falling due to age-related changes in their bodies, maintaining balance is essential for preventing falls. The following are the main points emphasizing the significance of balance in preventing falls:

- **Lowers The Risk Of Falls:**

  Seniors who have good balance are less likely to fall. It enables people to maintain stability when engaging in a variety of activities, including walking, standing, and even reaching for objects. The likelihood of losing control and falling significantly increases when balance is impaired.

- **Improves Posture And Body Alignment**:

Seniors with good balance are better able to keep their bodies aligned and maintain good posture, which eases the load on their muscles and joints.

- **Strengthen Muscles And Joints:**

Maintaining balance involves a mix of strength, coordination, and flexibility, all of which are crucial for preserving the health of muscles and joints. 3. Strengthens muscles and joints. Fall risk can be decreased by regularly performing balancing exercises that serve to strengthen the lower body, the core, and the joints.

- **Increases Mobility And Independence**:

  Seniors can increase their mobility and independence by concentrating on balance. A person with good balance can move with confidence and go about their everyday tasks without worrying about falling, such as ascending stairs, getting in and out of chairs, or walking on uneven terrain.

- **Boosts Confidence And Mental Well-being:** Fall-related injuries can have a significant impact on a person's confidence and mental well-being. Fear of falling can limit seniors' engagement in social activities, physical exercise, and even their ability to carry out routine tasks independently.

  By improving balance and reducing the risk of falls, seniors can regain

confidence and maintain a positive
outlook on their overall well-being.

- **Implements Fall Prevention Strategies:**

Focusing on balance provides an opportunity to implement fall prevention strategies. This can include exercises specifically designed to enhance balance, installing grab bars in bathrooms, removing tripping hazards in the home environment, and wearing appropriate footwear. All these measures contribute to a holistic approach towards fall prevention.

6.2 BALANCE EXERCISES FOR SENIORS:

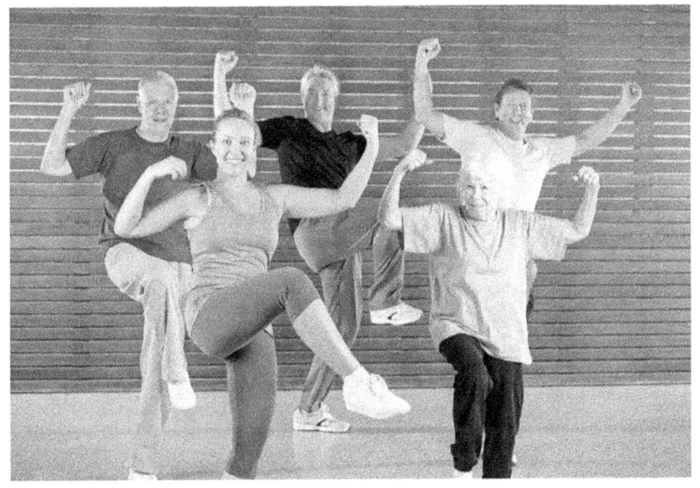

Yes, the following balancing drills can be helpful for seniors:

- **One-Legged Stance:**

  Take a 20- to 30-second stance on one leg before switching to the other. If necessary, use a chair or a wall as support.

- **Walk in a straight line:**

  While putting the toes of both feet together as you do a heel-to-toe motion

- **Leg Swings:**

  While holding onto a firm surface, swing one leg in front of and behind you, as well as from side to side. Continue with the opposite leg.

- **Tai Chi:**

  This gentle workout that includes deep breathing and flowing movements helps increase balance and flexibility. Standing

- **Yoga Poses :**

  Poses like the tree pose or the warrior pose can enhance balance and strength.

- **Marching In Place:**

  Raise each knee separately, switching between the legs, as though you were marching.

- **Side Leg Raises:**

  For balance, hold onto a chair and raise one leg out to the side before bringing it back in. Continue with the opposite leg.

- **Ankle Circles:**

  Rotate your ankle in a circular pattern while seated, lifting one foot off the floor. Change to your other foot.

- **Tandem Walk:**

  As if you were walking a tightrope, put one foot in front of the other.

- **Balance Board:**

  To challenge your balance in a controlled way, use a balance board or wobble cushion.

Never forget the necessity of placing safety first. Perform these exercises on a strong chair or wall nearby for support.

6.3 INTEGRATING BALANCE WORK INTO DAILY ACTIVITIES

A practical and efficient way to enhance balance and lower the chance of falling is to incorporate balance practice into regular activities. People can improve their balance abilities and maintain stability in a variety of scenarios by incorporating balance exercises into normal chores. The following are some strategies for including balance work in daily activities:

- **Standing On One Leg While Doing Home Duties:**

  Try standing on one leg while doing activities like brushing your teeth, doing the dishes, or conversing on the phone. This easy workout improves the muscles necessary for maintaining stability while testing the body's capacity to maintain balance. Begin with brief periods and gradually extend the time as your balance becomes more stable.

- **Balancing While Watching Television Or While In Line At The Grocery Shop:**

When you find yourself watching television or in line at the grocery store while there are commercial breaks, take use of the time to practice your balance. Try doing a tandem stand, which involves putting one foot in front of the other. These exercises strengthen the muscles in the core and enhance balance.

- **Balance Exercises During Daily Walks:**

This is a great approach to increase stability and balance while taking daily walks and enjoying the outdoors. Include actions that test the body's response to balance, such as heel-toe walking, side steps, or stepping over obstacles. To further improve balance, you might add walking on unlevel surfaces like gravel or grass.

- **Using balance aids during everyday tasks:**

  You can add a new level of challenge to your daily activities by including balance aids like stability balls, wobble boards, or balance cushions. For instance, try standing on a balancing cushion while cooking or sitting on a stability ball while watching television. These tools help to strengthen the core muscles and control balance.

- **Choosing to use the stairs rather than the elevator:**

  Choosing to use the stairs is a great way to incorporate balance work into daily living. Because it calls for balance and coordination, stairs is a natural way to develop strong leg muscles and activate the body's balancing systems. As your fitness and balance improve, start with a few flights of stairs and progressively increase the distance.

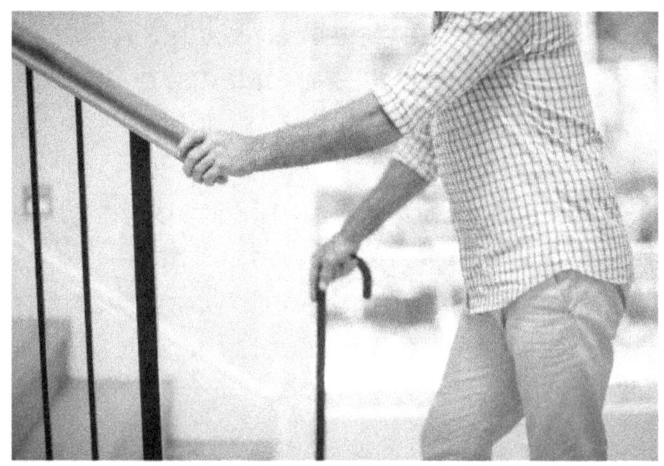

CHAPTER 7

MAINTAINING FLEXIBILITY AND MOBILITY

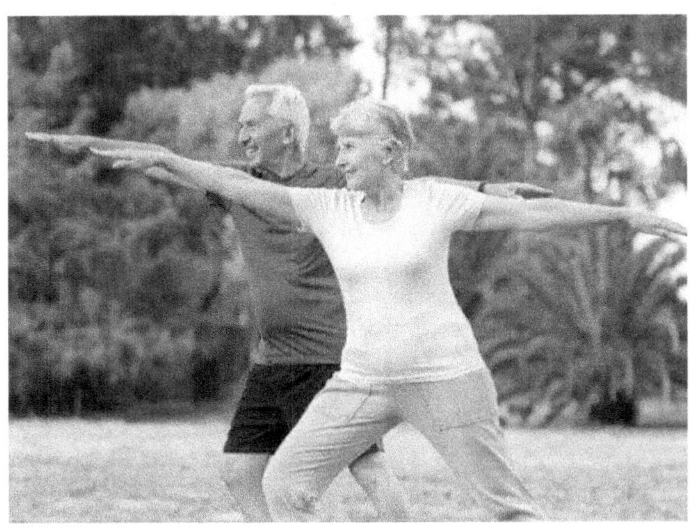

For general health and well-being, it's important to maintain mobility and flexibility. It entails maintaining joint mobility, avoiding muscle imbalances or tension, and keeping the body flexible. Regular mobility and stretching exercises can aid with flexibility, athletic performance, injury prevention, and better posture.

Additionally, preserving flexibility and mobility can benefit from including exercises like yoga, Pilates, or tai chi into one's routine. Stretching and mobility exercises should be prioritized as part of a comprehensive fitness program to enhance overall physical health.

7.1 GENTLE STRETCHING ROUTINES FOR SENIORS

Here are a few gentle stretching routines suitable for seniors.

- **Neck Stretch:**

  Gently tilt your head to the right, bringing your ear towards your shoulder. Hold for 15-20 seconds, then switch sides.

- **Shoulder Roll:**

  Roll your shoulders in a circular motion, first forward for 10 seconds, then backward for 10 seconds.

- **Arm Stretch:**

  Extend one arm out in front of you and gently pull it across your body with your other hand. Hold for 15-20 seconds, then switch arms.

- **Side Stretch:**

Stand or sit up straight, raise your right arm, and reach over to the left side. Hold for 15-20 seconds, then switch sides.

- **Quad Stretch:**

Hold onto a chair or wall for support. Bend one knee and gently grab your ankle, pulling it towards your glutes. Hold for 15-20 seconds, then switch legs.

- **Ankle Circles:**

Sit in a chair and raise one foot off the floor to perform ankle circles. Rotate your ankle for about 10 seconds in circles, first in one direction and then the other.

7.2 YOGA AND TAI CHI FOR FLEXIBILITY AND MINDFULNESS

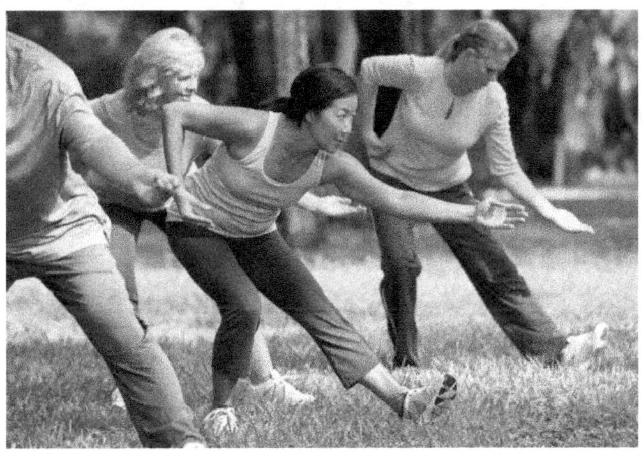

Two age-old disciplines, Yoga and Tai chi, provide many advantages for flexibility, mindfulness, and general well-being. These exercises combine fluid movements with deep breathing and meditation, which helps the body to stretch and strengthen while encouraging inner peace and focus.

Poses, or postures, are used in yoga to work on specific body areas. Yoga helps release tension in the muscles and joints, increase range of motion, and develop flexibility through a sequence of moderate stretches and holds. The benefits of regular yoga practice include better posture, fewer muscular imbalances, and increased coordination.

Overall, yoga and Tai Chi provide an all-encompassing strategy for preserving flexibility and mindfulness. People can gain physical, mental, and emotional advantages by implementing these activities into their daily routines, which will improve their overall health and well-being.

7.3 MIND-BODY CONNECTION:

The mind-body connection refers to the intricate and powerful link between our mental and emotional states and our physical well-being. It is the recognition that our thoughts, feelings, attitudes, and beliefs can profoundly affect our physical health and vice versa. Several practices and techniques can help strengthen the mind-body connection.

By acknowledging and nurturing the mind-body connection, we can become more aware of the impact our thoughts, emotions, and beliefs have on our physical health.

CHAPTER 8

ENGAGEMENT AND FUN ACTIVITIES

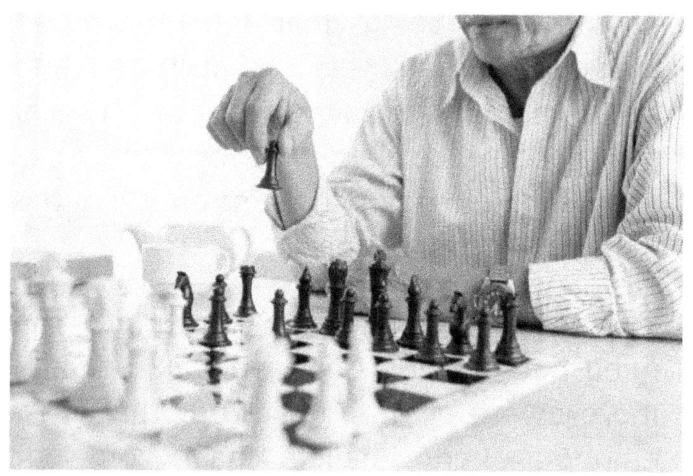

Fun activities are not only pleasurable, but also essential for senior citizens' general wellbeing. They can significantly improve their quality of life, increase cognitive function, and lower their risk of developing mental health conditions like depression and anxiety by engaging in activities that offer cerebral stimulation, physical activity, social connection, and a sense of purpose. The following are some entertaining activities for seniors:

- **Arts and crafts:**

   Encouraging seniors to express their creativity via painting, drawing, ceramics, knitting, or other craft endeavors can be a rewarding and entertaining pastime. They are able to express themselves artistically while developing cognitive abilities including focus, problem-solving, and fine motor skills.

- **Music Therapy:**

   Music has a strong emotional impact and can significantly raise one's spirits. Seniors can benefit greatly by participating in music-related activities, such as singing, playing musical instruments, or simply listening to their favorite music. It can enhance mood, jog memory, and evoke feelings of connection and nostalgia.

- **Gentle Exercise:**

It's important to stay physically active to keep your body healthy and mobile. Stretching, chair yoga, or tai chi are examples of easy exercises that can help seniors keep active and preserve their strength, flexibility, and balance. Senior-specific group exercise courses can help promote social contact and a sense of community.

- **Games And Puzzles:**

Seniors who want to keep their wits active and sharp should engage in board games, card games, riddles, and brainteasers. Games like chess, Scrabble, Sudoku, or jigsaw puzzles provide fun social interactions with friends or family while also providing opportunity to practice memory, problem-solving, and strategic thinking skills.

- **Outdoor Activities:**

Being outside gives elders the chance to get in touch with nature and take in some sunshine and fresh air. Gardening, nature walks, bird watching, and park picnics are a few examples of activities that can be wonderfully reviving and energizing. It has been demonstrated that spending time in nature lowers stress, boosts mood, and enhances general wellbeing.

8.1 GROUP FITNESS CLASSES AND CLUBS

People can work out together in creative and inspiring ways through group fitness courses and clubs. Numerous exercises are frequently included in these programs, including yoga, spinning, HIIT, and others. They offer a regimented setting, qualified direction, and the companionship of exercising with others, which can increase motivation and accountability. Group fitness is a popular option for individuals looking for both physical activity and social interaction because it can accommodate different fitness levels and goals.

8.2 Dancing, Walking, and Outdoor Activities

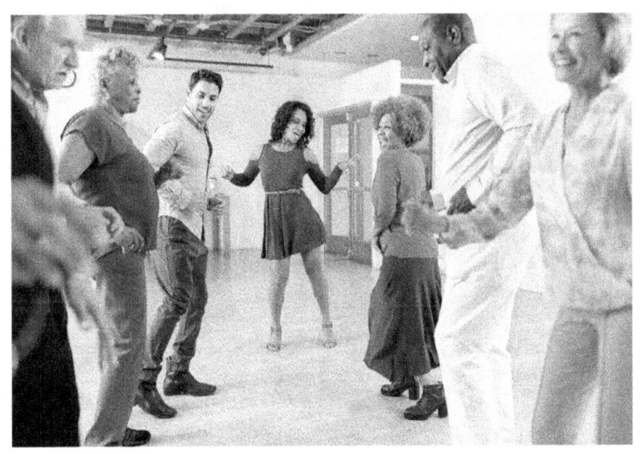

- **Dancing**

  is a fun and expressive art form as well as a pleasurable form of exercise. Whether you dance to the rhythm in a ballroom, hip-hop, salsa, or contemporary style, you can engage every muscle in your body. Dancing improves coordination, flexibility, and cardiovascular fitness while also releasing endorphins, which improve mood.

It's a fantastic way to interact with others, decompress, and enhance general physical wellness.

- **Walking**:

People of all ages and fitness levels can benefit from this low-impact but very effective type of exercise. It can be incorporated into daily routines and doesn't require any specialized equipment. Walking quickly can develop your muscles, boost your cardiovascular health, and aid in weight loss. Additionally, because it has a minimal impact, it lowers the possibility of joint strain.

- **Outdoor Activities:**

Taking part in outdoor activities, like hiking, biking, and playing sports, has a number of positive effects on both physical and mental health. These activities, which can be done alone or in groups, combine physical activity with a love of nature. Hiking, for instance, offers a sense of adventure while taxing the body's muscles and cardiovascular system. Cycling increases cardiovascular fitness and leg strength. Team sports like soccer and volleyball encourage collaboration and socialization while also enhancing agility and coordination.

Overall, there are many different ways to maintain an active lifestyle, including dancing, walking, and outdoor hobbies. Finding activities that people enjoy and can stick with over time is made simpler by the variety of options available that appeal to diverse preferences and fitness levels.

8.3 CREATING A SUPPORTIVE FITNESS COMMUNITY

Fostering a welcoming environment where participants encourage and support one another in achieving their fitness objectives is essential to building a friendly fitness community. This can be accomplished through having open lines of communication, reporting on accomplishments, planning group activities, and showing support for both achievements and failures. Remember that creating a thriving fitness community requires a sense of community and support among members.

CHAPTER 9

OVERCOMING CHALLENGES AND STAYING MOTIVATED

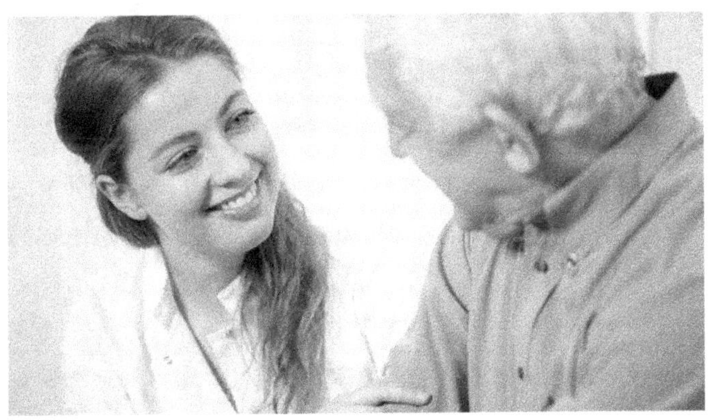

Several crucial techniques are required for seniors who want to achieve fitness freedom in order to overcome obstacles and maintain motivation. First, make goals that are appropriate for your ability and state of health. Even though progress could be delayed, persistence is what really counts. Keep in touch with a helpful network, whether it be friends, family, or other fitness aficionados. Participating in social interactions can offer support and accountability. Try a variety of exercises as well to keep things fresh and avoid getting bored. Keep in mind to pay attention to your body and modify as necessary. Prioritizing safety and avoiding excessive exertion are crucial. Before beginning any exercise program, it is advisable to speak with a healthcare practitioner.

Recognize that setbacks are common and enjoy tiny successes along the road. Since effects could take longer to manifest, patience is essential. Focus on the advantages of greater fitness and how they will improve your quality of life as a whole.

Finally, continue growing and changing. Keep an open mind to new tactics, exercises, and wellness rituals that are appropriate for you. You can achieve fitness freedom and keep your drive as you age by adopting a positive attitude and a gradual approach.

9.1 ADAPTING YOUR ROUTINE TO CHANGING ABILITIES

Here are some practical strategies for adapting your routine to changing abilities:

- **Evaluate Your Talents:**

To get a comprehensive picture of your existing capabilities, regularly evaluate your physical, cognitive, and emotional capacities. Tell yourself the truth about any obstacles or limits you may be facing.

- **Give Self-care Top Priority:**

Self-care is essential for preserving the best possible health and well-being. Find ways to take care of yourself, such as through exercise, a nutritious diet, enough sleep, and stress management. While still placing an emphasis on your physical and mental wellness, adapt these activities to fit your present level of ability.

- **Divide work into manageable steps:**

If you see that some chores are becoming more difficult, divide them into smaller, more manageable pieces. To make the procedure simpler, prepare dishes in bulk or use pre-cut and pre-packaged products if cooking a meal feels daunting. By doing this, you may still eat wholesome, home-cooked meals without putting an undue amount of physical or mental effort into them.

- **Modify your surroundings:**

Make changes to your living space to make it safe and accommodating of your evolving talents. This can entail adding grab bars to the bathroom, improving lighting throughout the house, reducing trip hazards, or shifting furniture around to make space for a wheelchair. Your safety and independence can be significantly improved with a few small changes.

- **Look For Social Support:**

Social interaction and solid relationships with family, friends, and neighbors are crucial for emotional well-being. Join senior centers, clubs, or neighborhood organizations that fit your interests and skills. These social connections can bring a sense of purpose and satisfaction in addition to support.

9.2 CELEBRATING ACHIEVEMENTS AND PROGRESS

"Cheers to Seniors' Fitness Freedom: Celebrating Achievements!

In the pursuit of fitness freedom, our seniors are shining examples of dedication and progress. Each step, each milestone they conquer is a testament to their determination and resilience. Their journey is a celebration of breaking barriers, redefining possibilities, and proving that age is no obstacle to vitality. Let's applaud their achievements and find inspiration in their remarkable progress."

CHAPTER 10

SAFETY TIPS FOR EXERCISING AT HOME

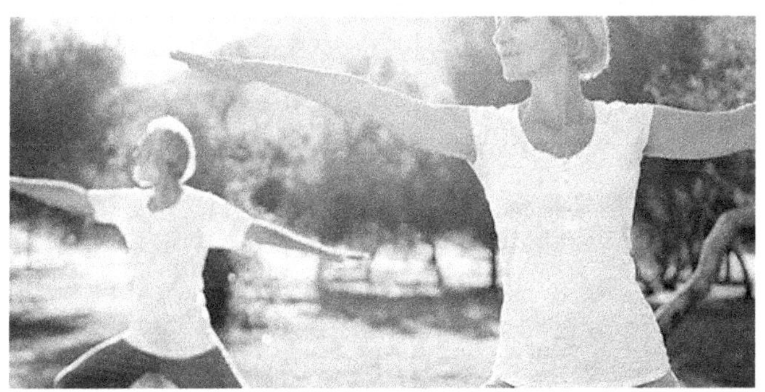

Recently, especially in light of the present pandemic, exercising at home has grown in popularity. However, it's crucial to follow the right safety precautions when working out at home to avoid accidents or injuries. Observe the following safety advice:

- **Warm-up and cool-down:**

Before starting any exercise program, it's vital to warm up your muscles and joints. This can help you progressively raise your heart rate and help you avoid accidents. In a similar vein, cooling off is crucial for gradually lowering your heart rate after activity. Additionally, cooling off can help stop fainting or dizziness.

- **Use the right equipment:**

Make sure any workout tools you use, such as jump ropes, resistance bands, or dumbbells, are in good working order. Look for any worn-out or broken components before use.

- **Pick a secure location:**

Pick a well-lit, secure place of your house to work out. Make sure there are no obstructions, kids, or pets in the area. To avoid slipping on hard surfaces when performing floor workouts, think about using a mat.

- **Keep your body hydrated:**

  By drinking plenty of water prior to, during, and after your workout. Dehydration can result in headaches, tiredness, and vertigo.

- **Adjust workouts:**

  Adjust exercises to your needs if you have existing injuries or medical concerns. Avoid any workout that hurts or makes you uncomfortable. For suggestions on the proper alterations, speak with your healthcare professional or a qualified trainer.

- **Dress appropriately:**

Put on loose-fitting, breathable clothing that is comfortable and allows you to move easily. Avoid wearing loose apparel that could trip you up or get trapped in equipment.

- **Pay attention to instructions**:

If you're using an exercise video or software, pay close attention to the directions. Exercises that are beyond your level of proficiency or that demand advanced abilities should not be attempted.

- **Be aware of your surroundings:**

Keep an eye out for any potential dangers and pay attention to your surroundings. Make sure you're not close to any sharp objects or walls, for instance, if you're using a stability ball..

- **Seek expert advice:**

For advice on safe and efficient workout regimens, think about seeking the advice of a licensed trainer or physical therapist.

They can offer advice on appropriate form, adjustments, and advancements.

In conclusion, exercising at home can be a secure and efficient way to maintain an active lifestyle, but it's crucial to put safety first. You may avoid injuries, enjoy your workout, and reach your fitness objectives by using the advice in this article.

10.1 FINDING PROFESSIONAL GUIDANCE AND RESOURCES

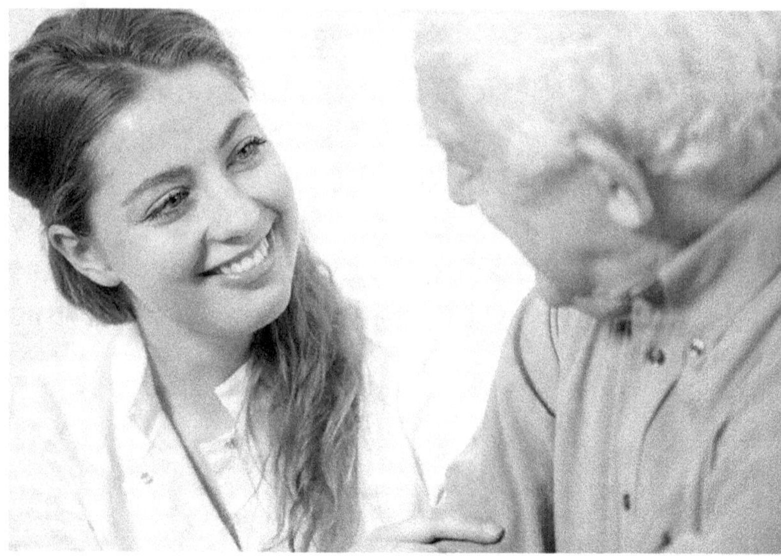

You can find professional guidance and resources for through various avenues:

- **Certified Trainers and Physical Therapists:**

  Look for physical therapists or trainers who have experience dealing with senior citizens. Based on specific demands and medical situations, they can offer tailored advice.

- **Local gyms and community centers:**

  A lot of local gyms and centers in the community provide senior fitness classes or programs. Senior-specific requirements are frequently catered to by instructors in these situations.

- **Senior Centers:**

  Take advantage of the fitness courses and other activities that are frequently offered in your neighborhood senior centers.

- **Online materials:**

Senior fitness materials are available on a variety of websites and online communities, including guidelines, articles, and training videos. The National Institute on Aging, AARP, and SilverSneakers are a few examples.

- **Healthcare Providers:**

Before starting any new exercise regimen, speak with your healthcare physician. They can make suggestions and guarantee that the exercises you choose are appropriate for your level of health.

- **Fitness Apps:**

Some fitness apps offer routines that can be done at home or at a gym and are tailored for older people.

Utilize social media to keep up with fitness professionals and businesses that offer senior-specific routines and guidance.

- **Books and Publications:**

 Look for publications that are devoted to senior fitness; they might offer insightful advice.

BONUS!!!: TIPS FOR WEAKER AND OLD AGE PEOPLE

If you are a senior citizen and striving for good health then, this chapter will

give you perfect ways to maintain a very fit and healthy body.

- Keep your mind young
- Some secret health tips for older people
- Regular health check ups
- Overcome your bad habits
- Senior safety at home

Our body is similar to an extremely fragile mechanism, and the more we use it, the more susceptible it is to malfunctions. Similar circumstances apply to aging since we have used practically all of our body's resources by the time we reach old age, necessitating particular care and close monitoring to keep it healthy and operating at full capacity. If you are in your early 40s, you should be aware that you are approaching an age where little illnesses could overwhelm you and leave you defenseless. Fortunately, there are many things you can do to enhance your daily life and maintain your fitness well into old age.

Keep Your Mind Young

Most people age because they believe they are already past their prime. Your state of mind has a profound impact on your general health. Never tell yourself that you are getting old and frail because if you did, it would only make you feel older and weaker.

You should remain positive and tell yourself that now is not the time to relax on your bed but rather to engage fully in daily activities. When they reach their fifties and have grandchildren, I've seen individuals lay down on their beds. This is not how it should be done; instead, you should continue to be involved and make an effort to do so in your family's affairs.

Some Secret Health Tips For Older People

Any age group can stay fit with regular exercise, but the types of exercise are always evolving. When you are young and healthy, you can afford to practice weightlifting, aerobics, and other similar workouts, but as you turn 50, your bones and muscles start to deteriorate, making it impossible for you to carry out all of those exercise regimens. You should be aware of this fact and select some easy and gentle exercises for yourself, such as stretching, walking, light jogging, and other activities. Walking and jogging are two of the most important and beneficial workouts you can do, and they will not only help you to maintain your health but also enable you to get rid of certain cardiac conditions and lung diseases.

You can also try light kinds of aerobics and other hard stretching exercise but try them for a particular period and see their effect. If you feel strain or pain in your muscles and weakness in your whole body then, you should know that these are not the appropriate exercises for you.

Regular Health Check ups:

As I mentioned above that in older age, your muscles, bones and other vital organs become weaker and they tend to get diseased and faulty very easily. So to avoid any unpleasant situation, you should have regular checkups from your doctor. These checkups will ensure that everything is working properly inside your body and even if something is going wrong, it will be diagnosed in early stages and doctors will be able to give you proper medication to cure it as soon as possible.

There is no better person thanyour family doctor to do this checkup because he knows your history and he will know your problems much better than a new doctor.

Overcome Your Bad Habit

As we get older, we pick up unhealthy habits like smoking, drinking, and other related activities. These behaviors may not be very harmful to you when you are young, and you will be able to withstand their negative consequences for your health at that age. However, when you get older, these behaviors may endanger your life.

At that age, drinking upsets your immune system, and you are no longer able to fend off its ill effects. Your digestive system may be destroyed, and it may also cause serious liver disorders. In a similar vein, smoking excessively can harm your lungs. You need to stop these habits if you want to make the remaining few years of your life easier on yourself.

If you can't quit them, then try to limit them.

Senior Safety At Home

In old age, people tend to fell sick a lot more often and it is necessary that they should be provided with proper support at home. Muscles become weak and sometime weakness becomes terrible and they cannot even walk properly.

In this condition, individuals require adequate support when ascending stairs, as well as adequate support in their bathrooms to prevent slips from the bathroom's slippery flooring. Going to an old-age home is not a great idea because it is undesirable from many angles. These areas have an extremely lonely atmosphere that disturbs your mental health. You always need family members to help you out and take care of you in your later years, especially your children. If someone you love is constantly there to support you during difficult times, it creates an atmosphere that is very calming and supportive.

11. EMBRACING A LIFELONG JOURNEY OF FITNESS FREEDOM

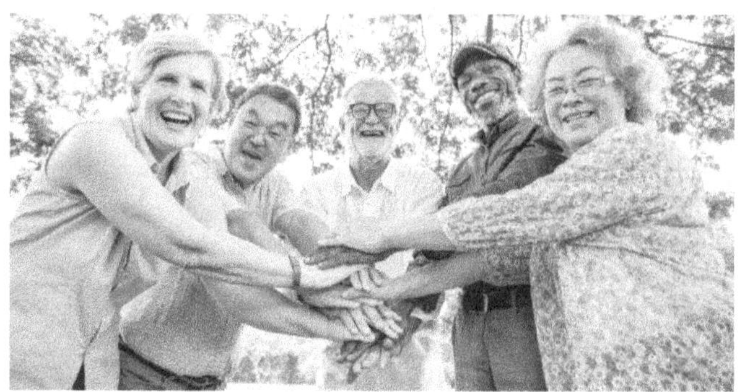

Adopting a Lifelong Journey of Fitness Freedom" entails committing to a healthy lifestyle that is sustainable and well-balanced. It's about fueling your body, enjoying activity, and adjusting to life's changes. Remember that this is your individual journey; enjoy each step and bask in the empowerment that comes with taking charge of your health.

CONCLUSION

Embracing fitness freedom for elders is a revolutionary approach to overall wellbeing; it goes beyond simply encouraging physical activity. Seniors can empower themselves to live a life full of vitality, vigor, and happiness by realizing that age is not a barrier. Seniors can overcome the limitations of aging and begin a meaningful journey of fitness by engaging in customized workouts, mindful eating, and a positive mindset. This journey isn't only about the body; it's about having the freedom to live life to the fullest, enjoying each moment of better health and increased vigor while also appreciating every accomplishment. Seniors' fitness freedom is proof of the human spirit's tenacity and the limitless opportunities that come with living a life of wellness

www.ingramcontent.com/pod-product-compliance
Lightning Source LLC
Chambersburg PA
CBHW050918260726

48660CB00001B/278